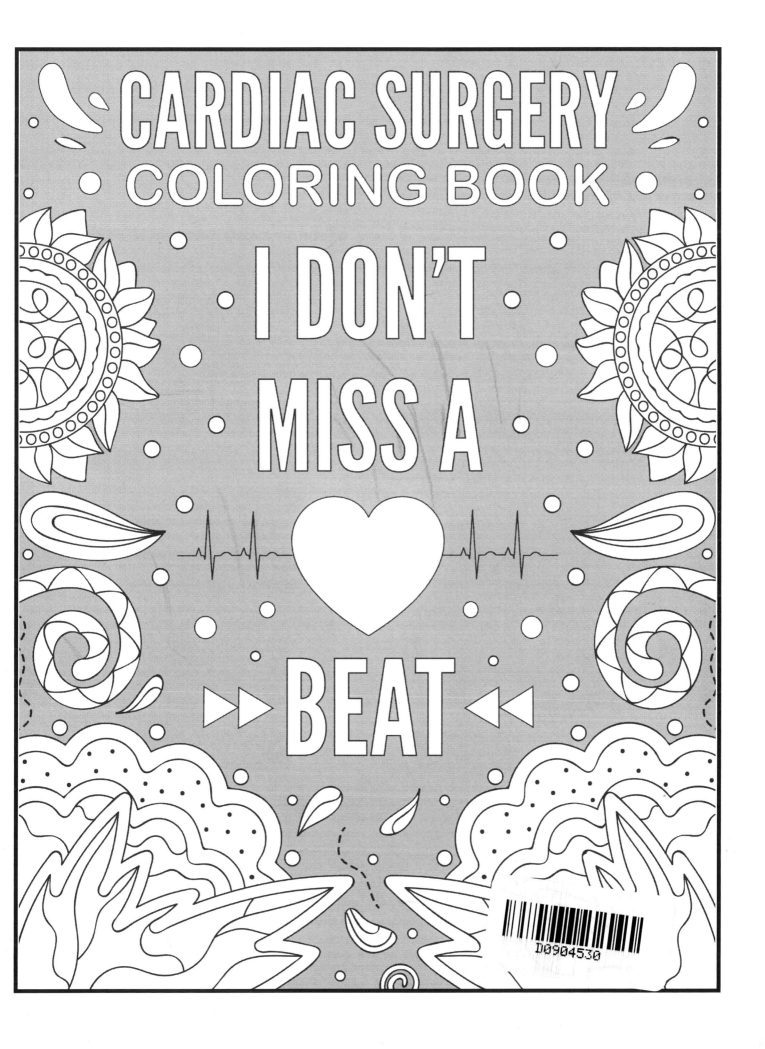

We would like to thank you personally for purchasing this book. This coloring book is a collection of funny and relatable Heart Surgery Coloring Pages.

At Gobisharad Sharmaji Publishing we understand that having a Heart surgery can be tough. So, to let you add some fun and relaxation to your Knee surgery recovery we have created this coloring book.

Published by Gobisharad Sharmaji Publishing

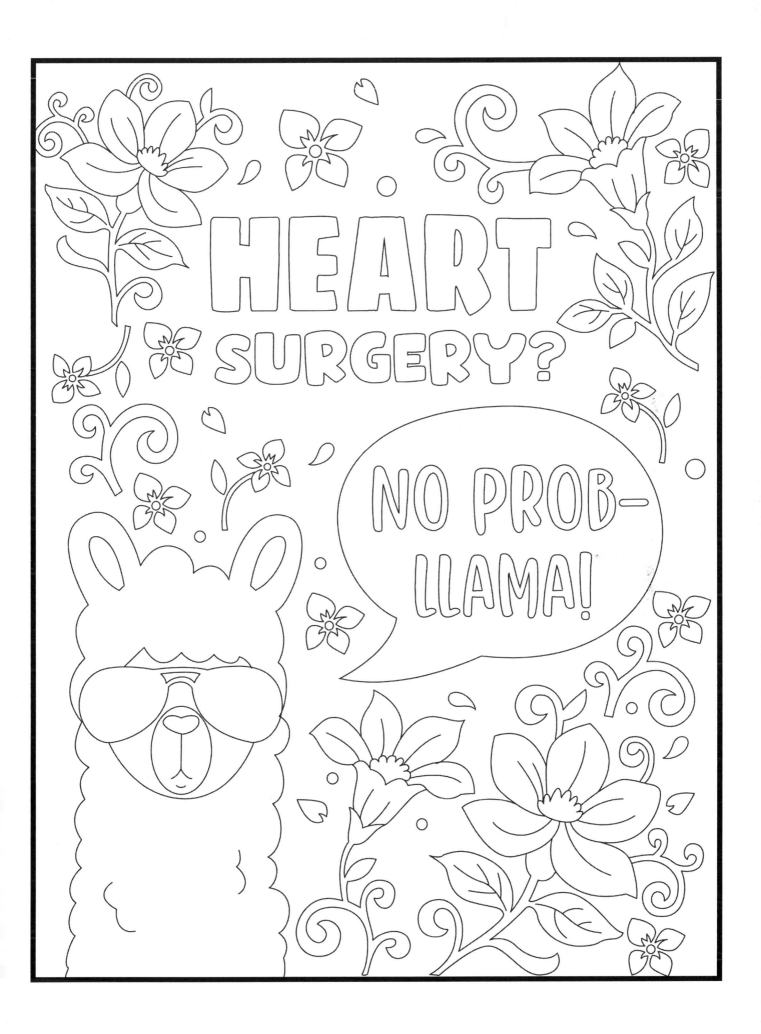

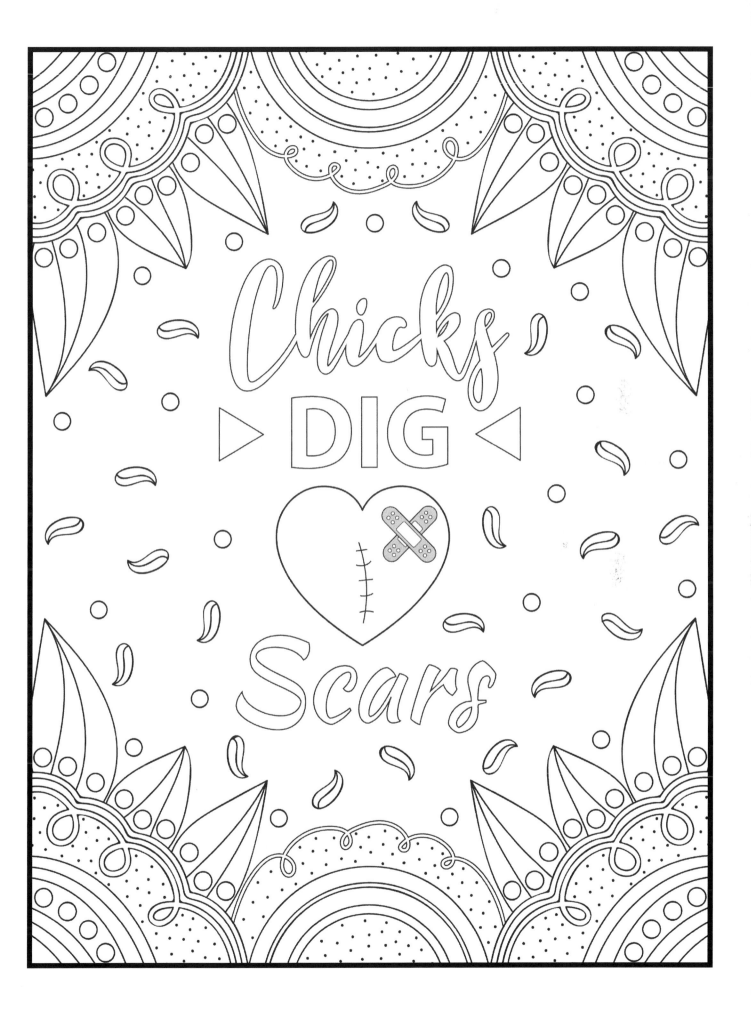

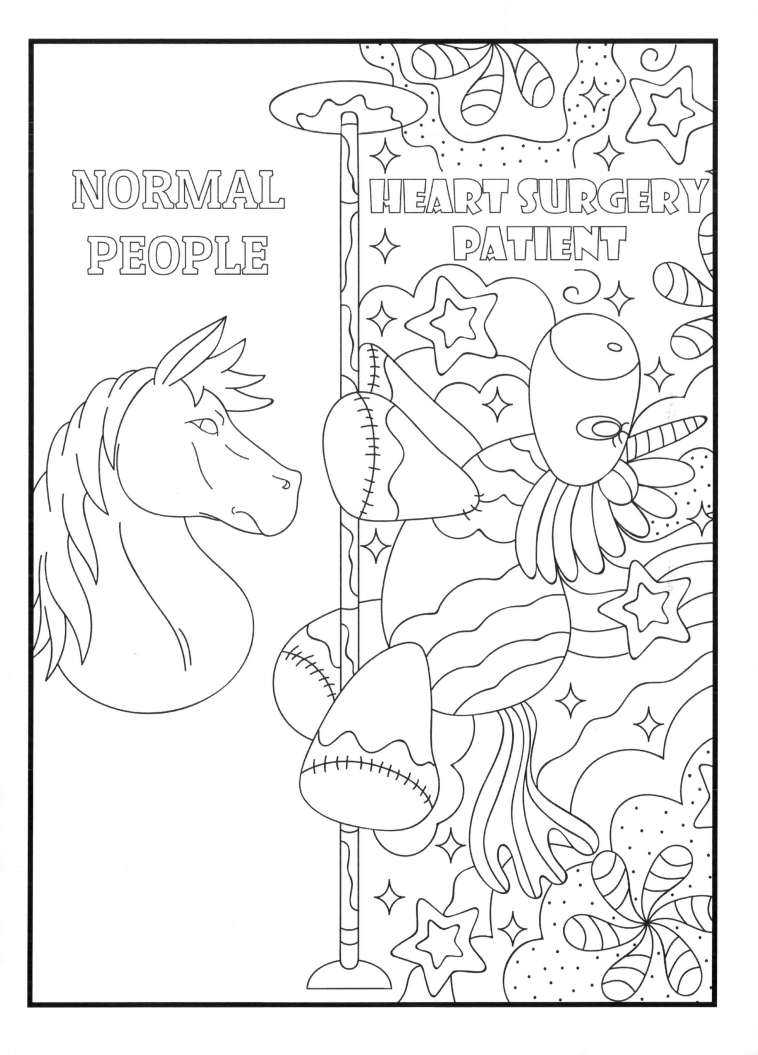

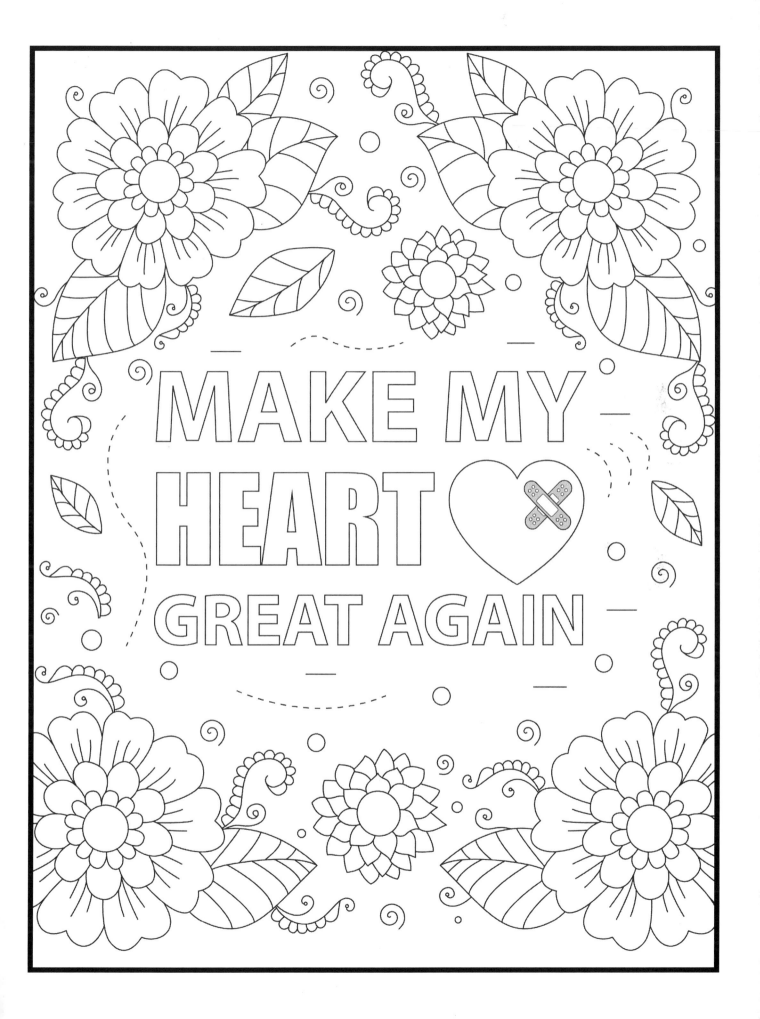

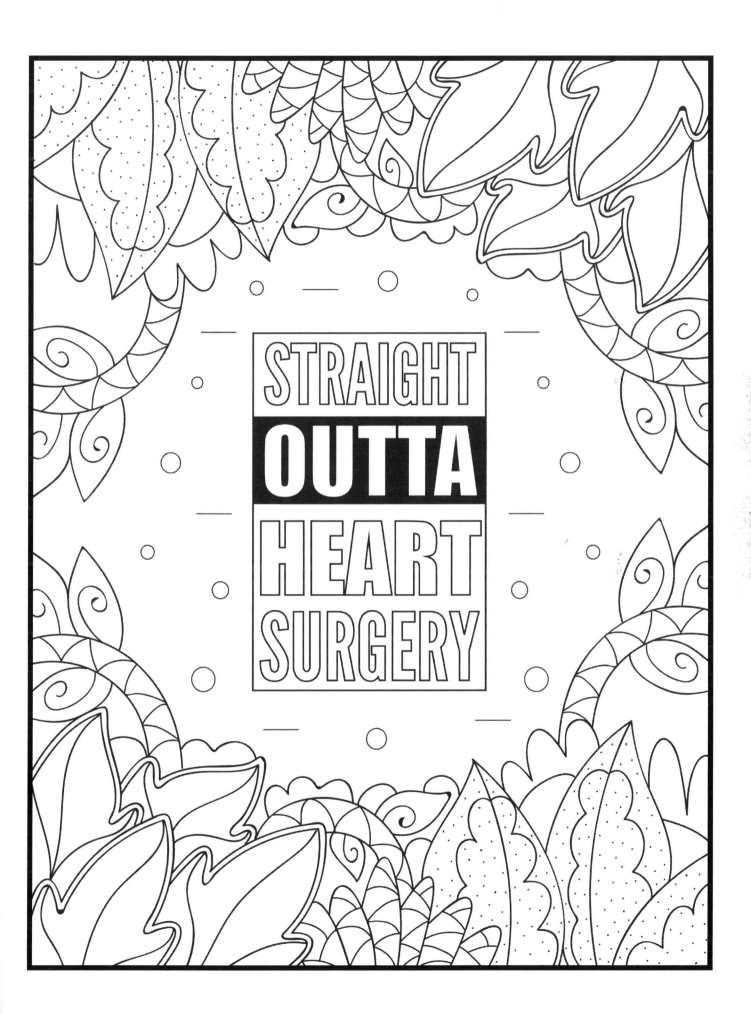

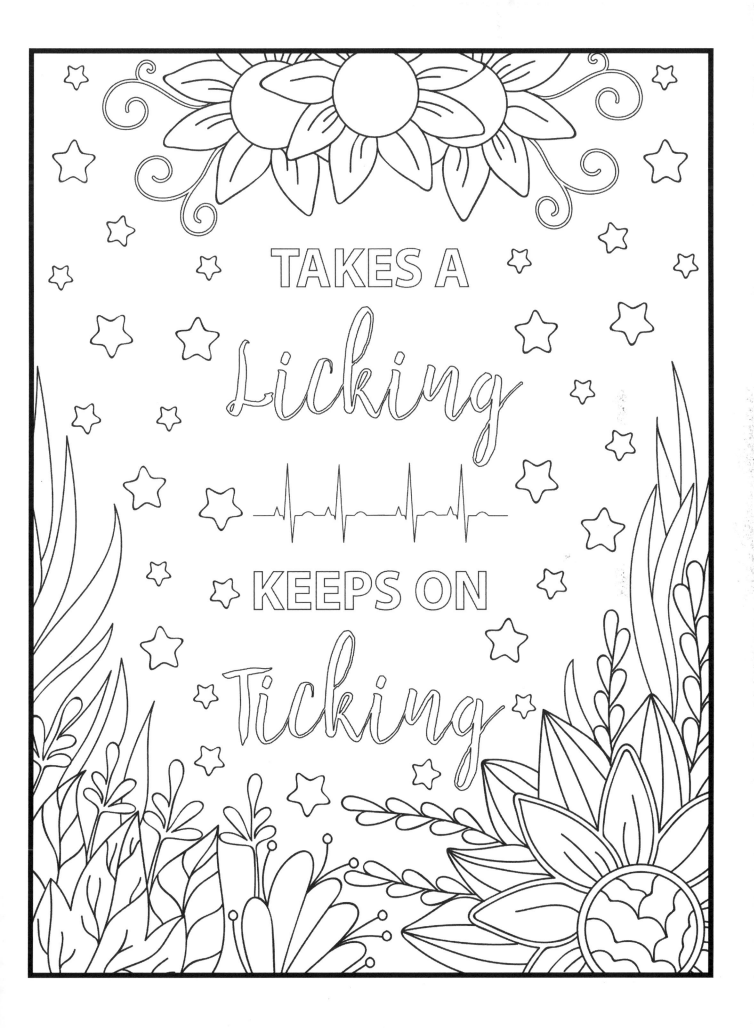

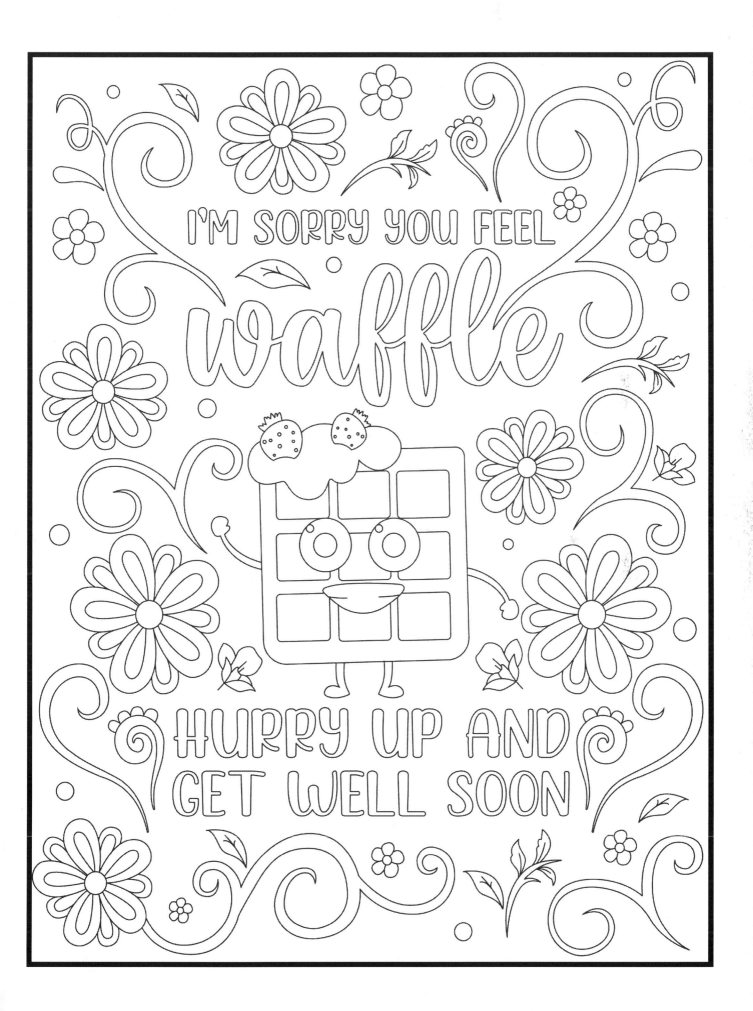

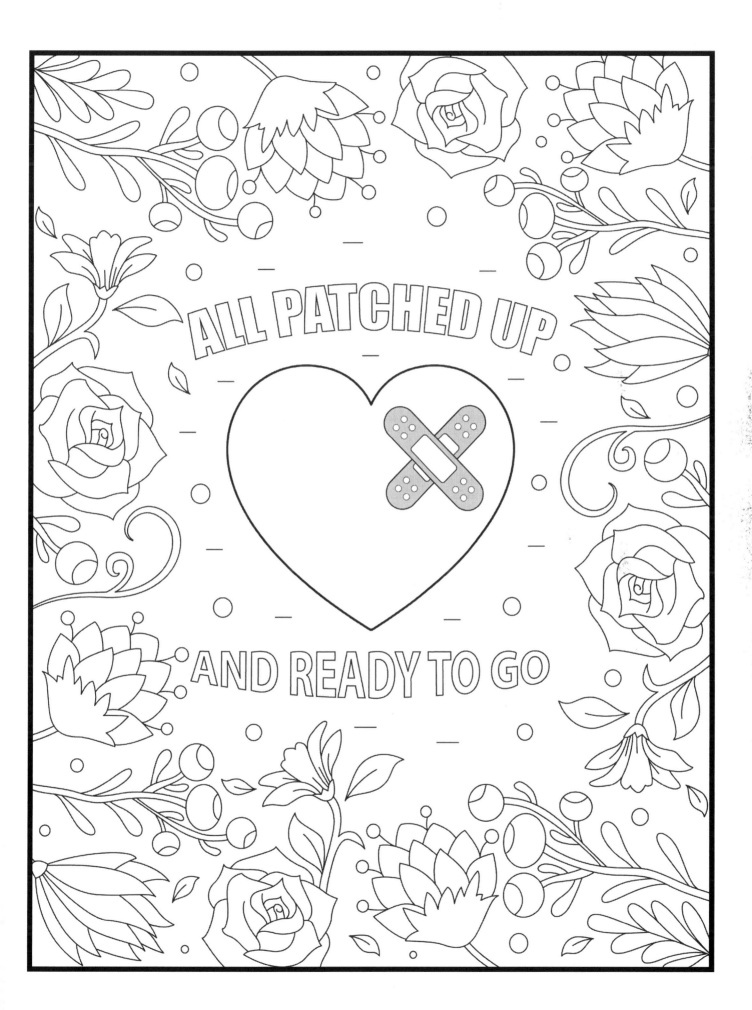

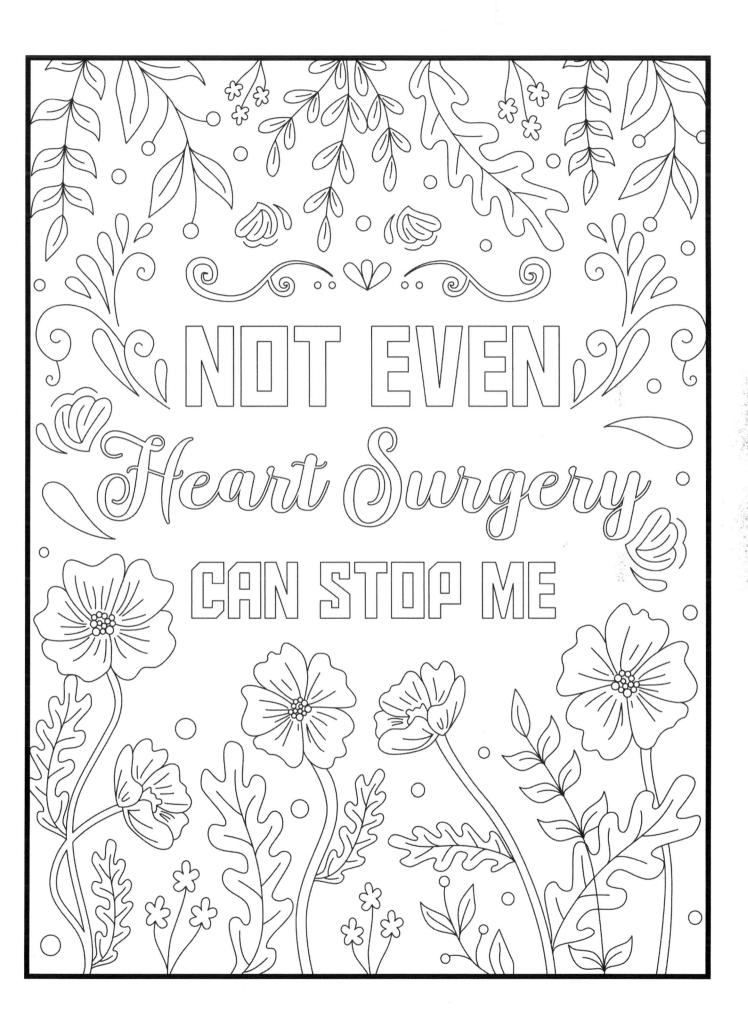

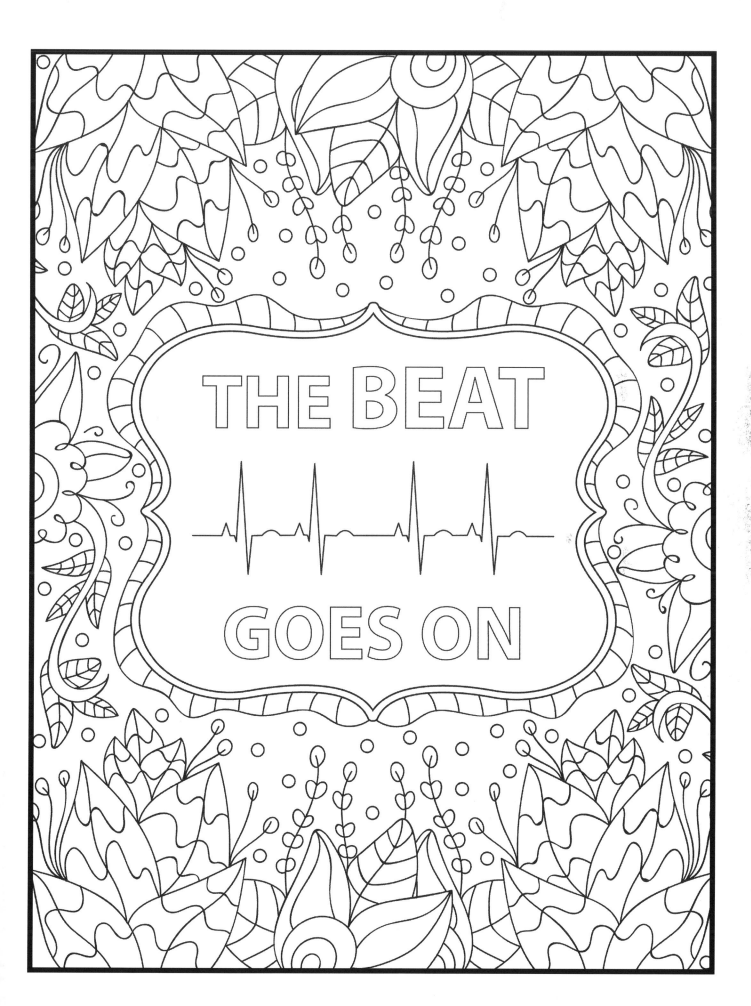

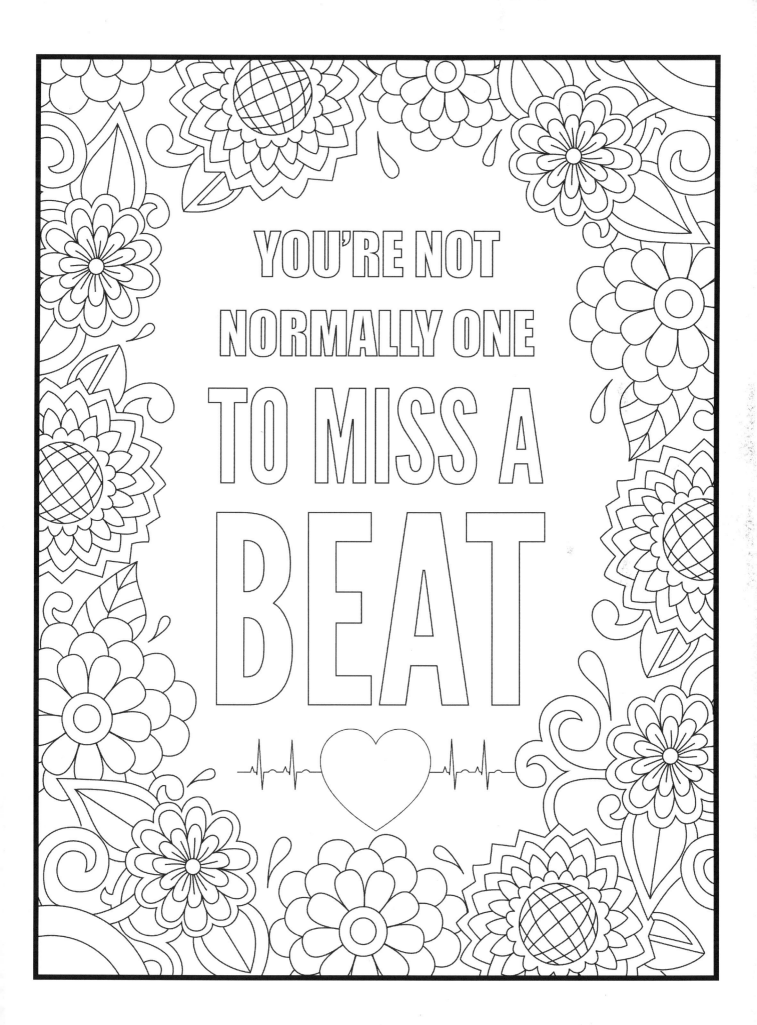

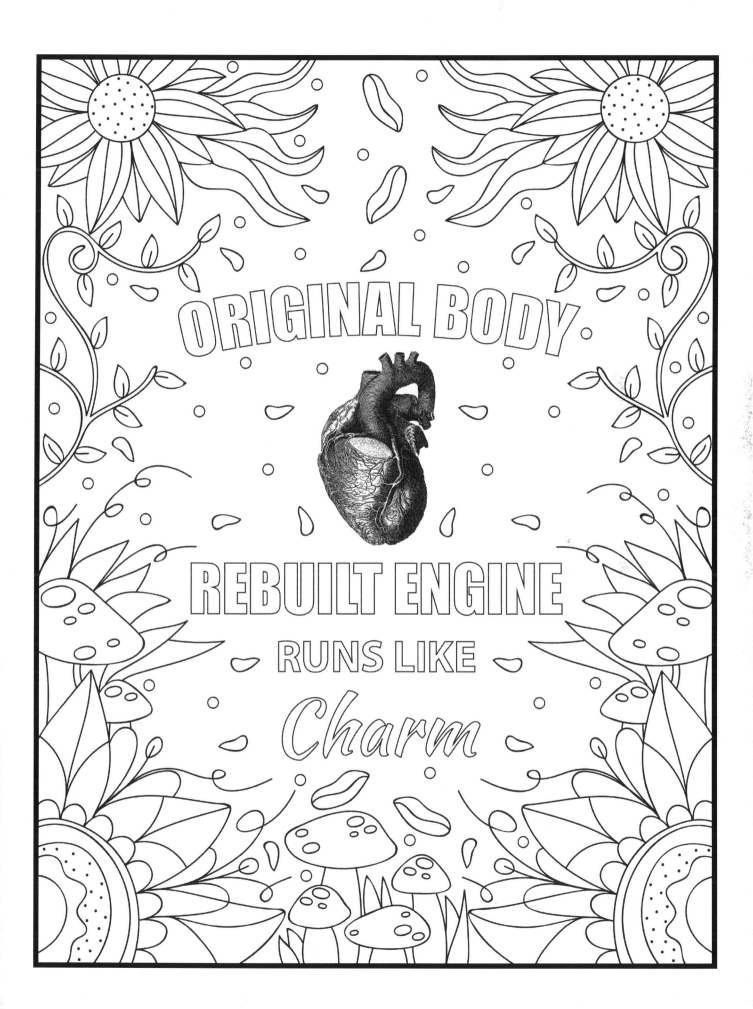

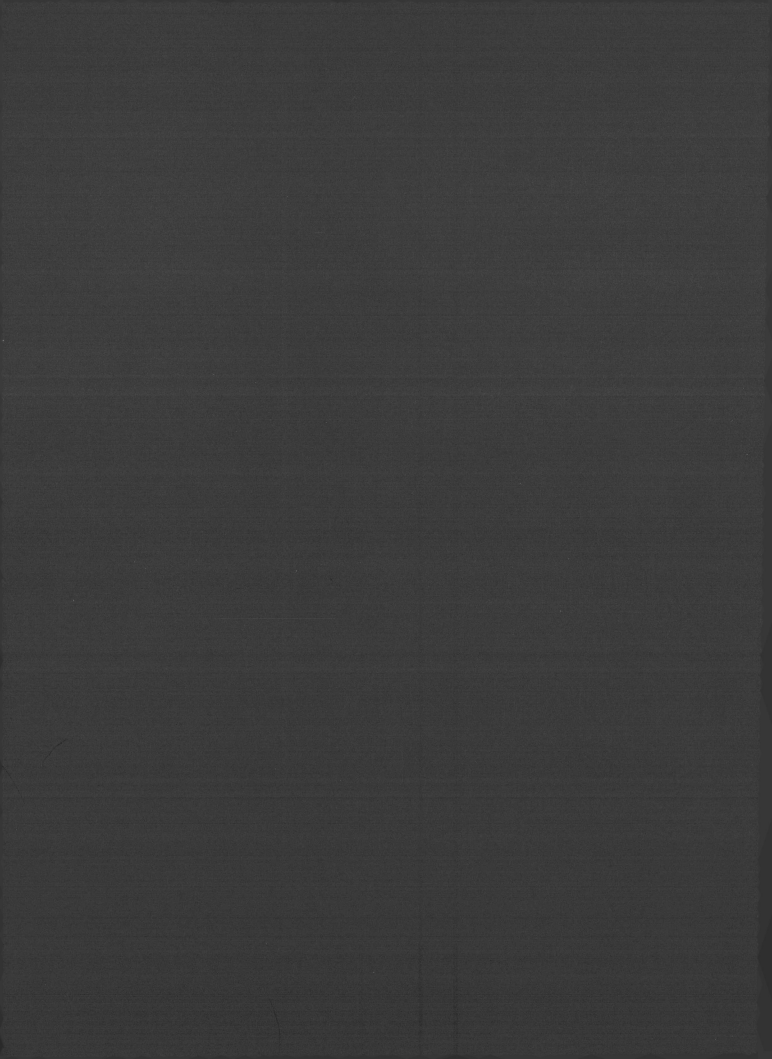

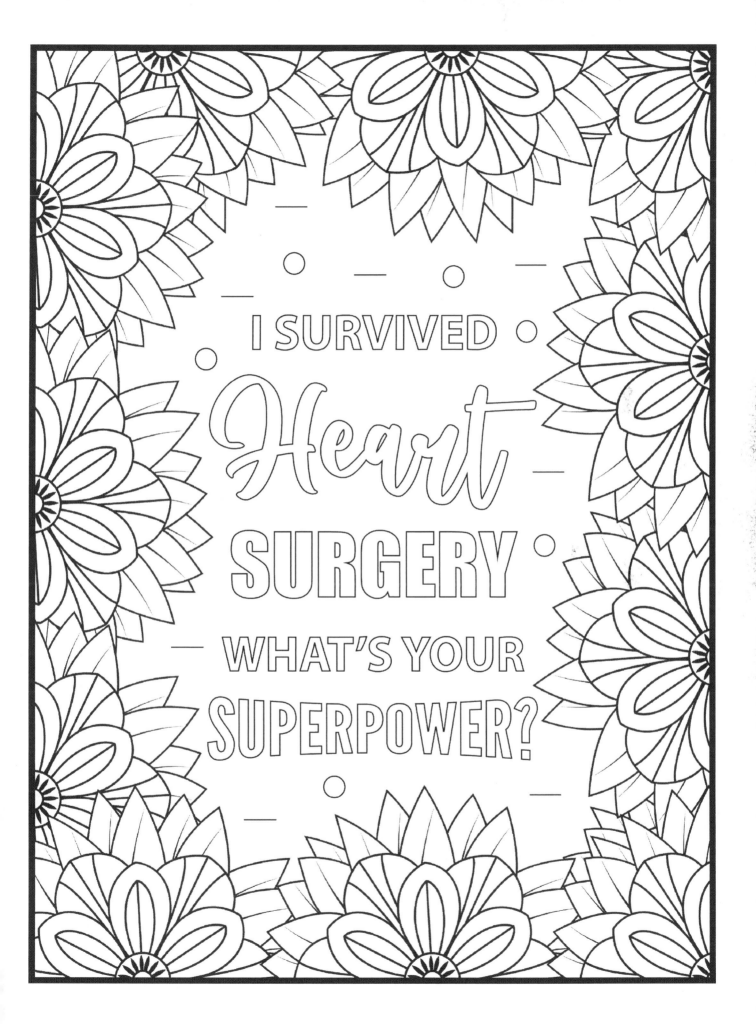

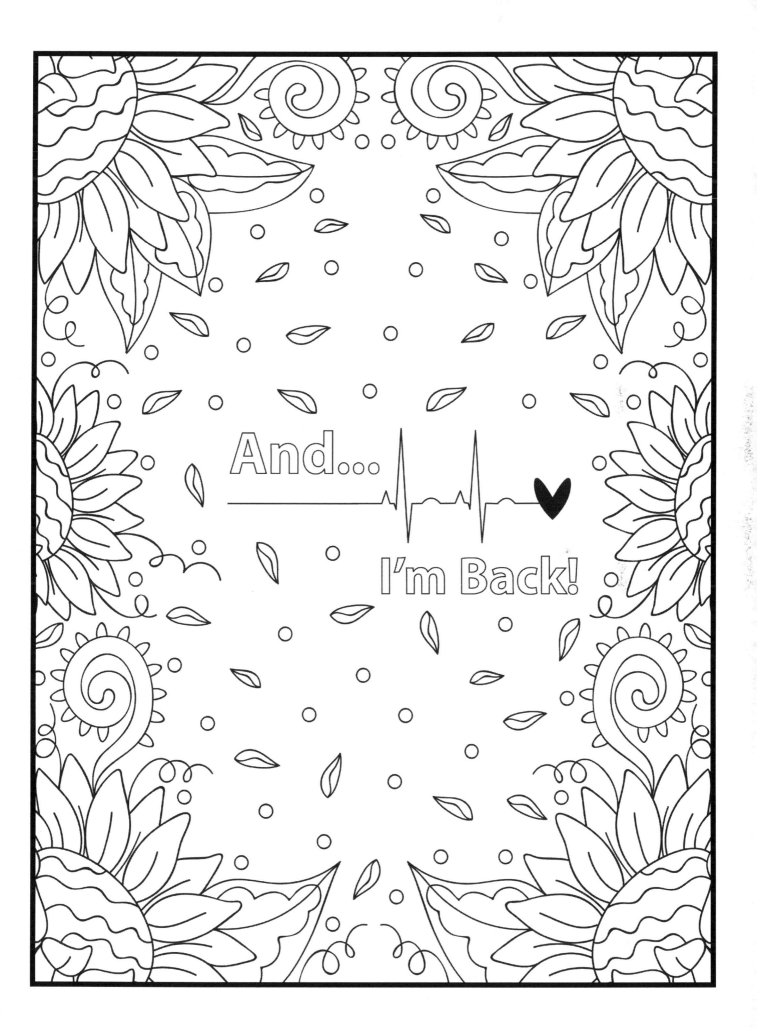

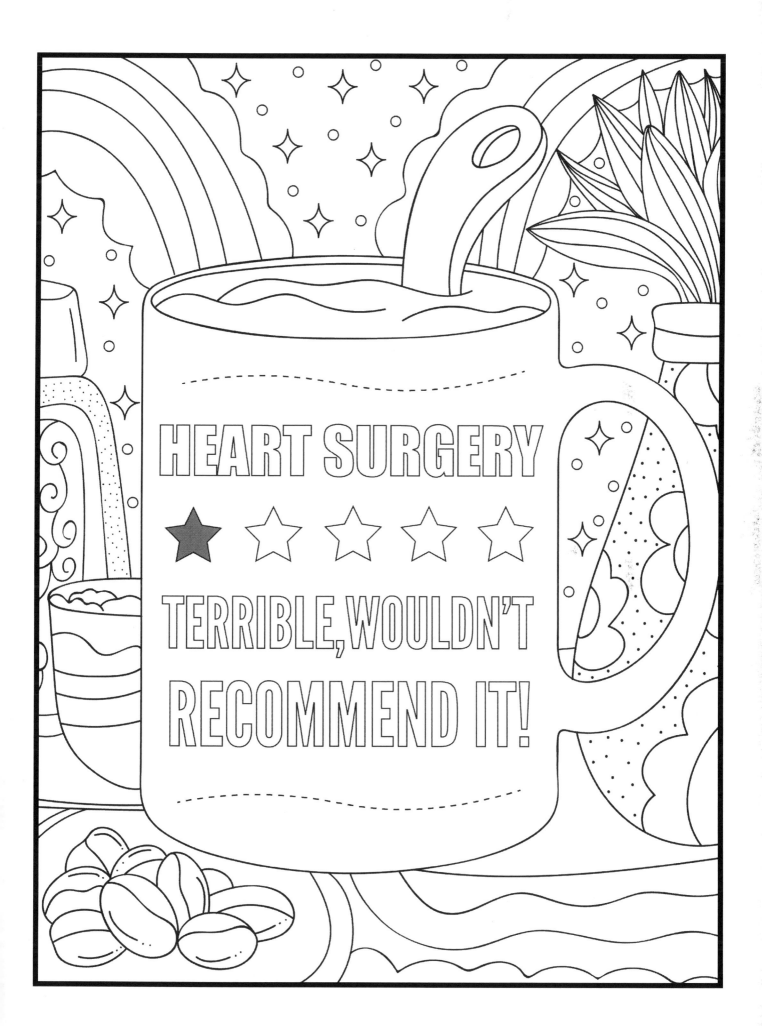

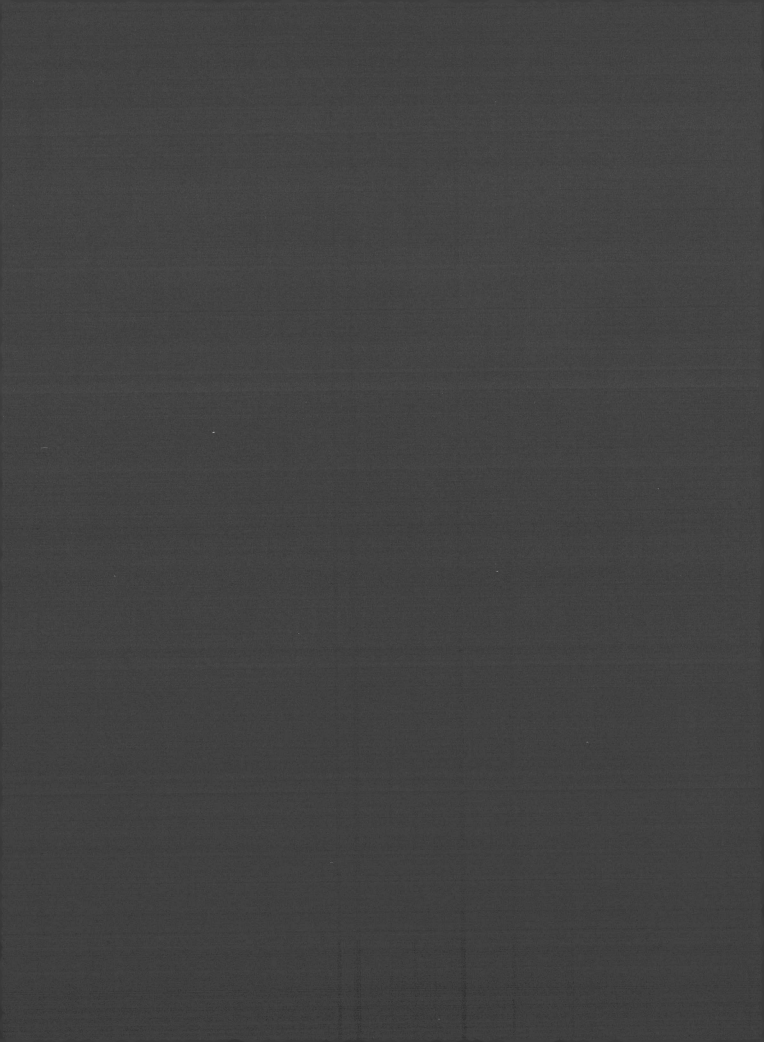

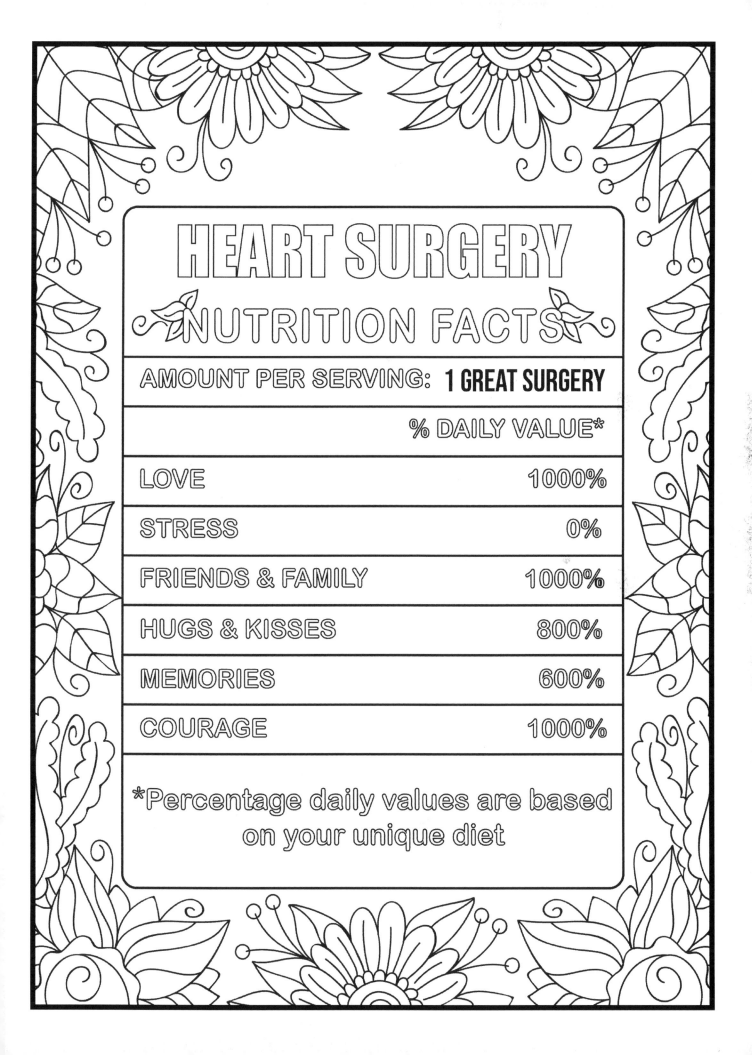

HEART SURGERY
NUTRITION FACTS

AMOUNT PER SERVING: **1 GREAT SURGERY**

% DAILY VALUE*

LOVE	1000%
STRESS	0%
FRIENDS & FAMILY	1000%
HUGS & KISSES	800%
MEMORIES	600%
COURAGE	1000%

*Percentage daily values are based on your unique diet

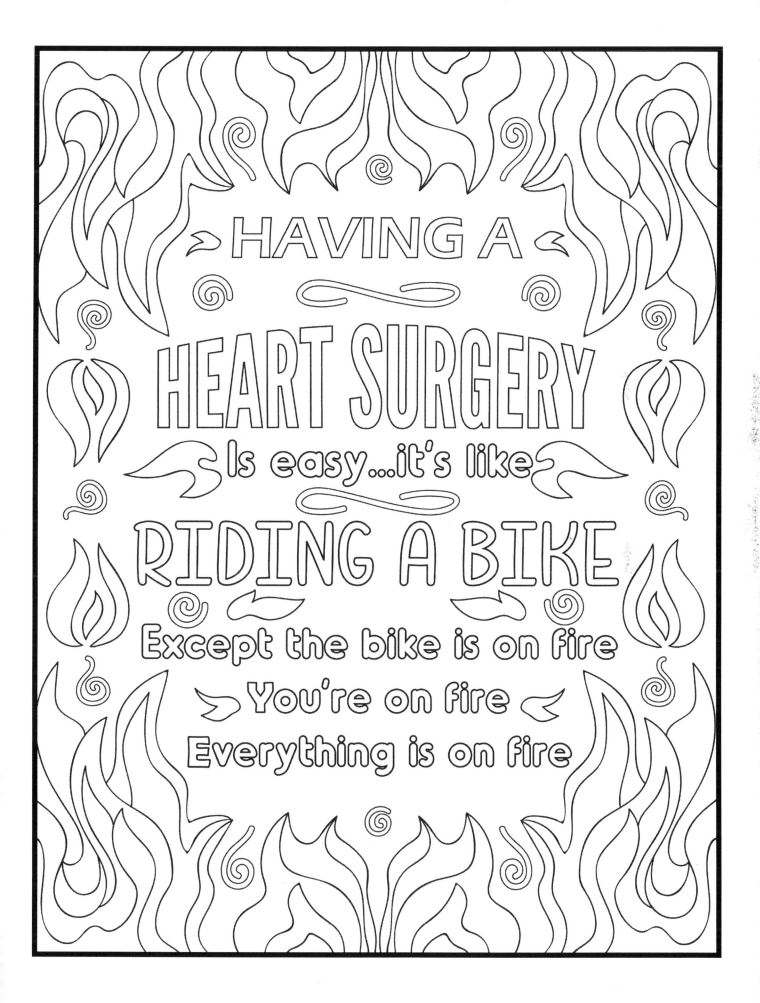

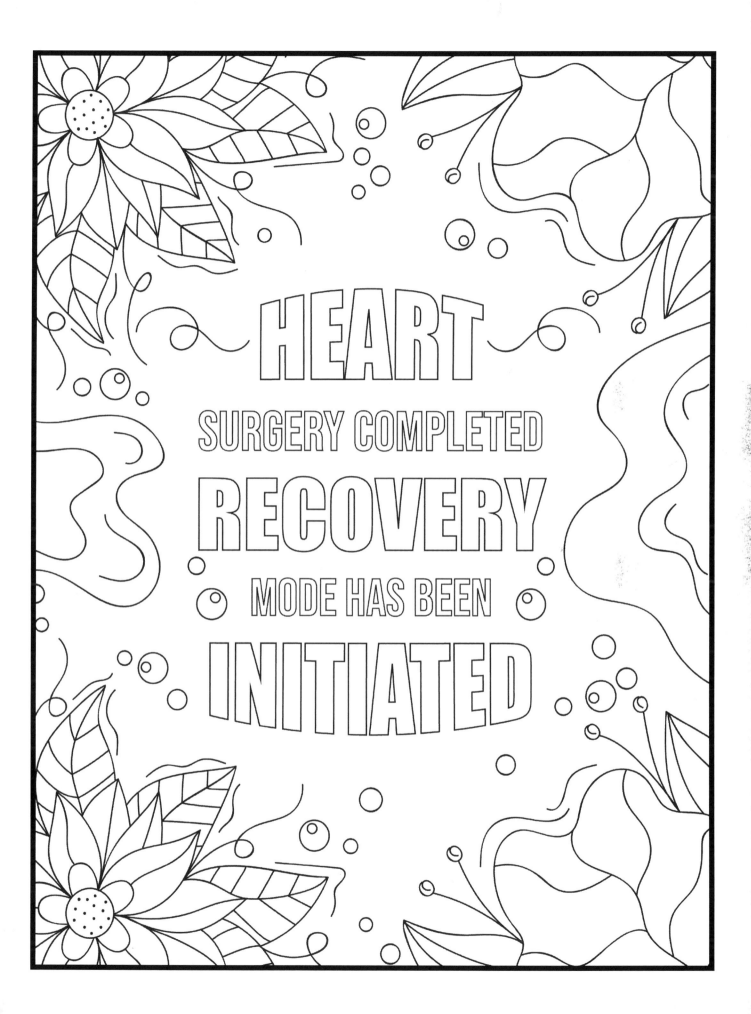

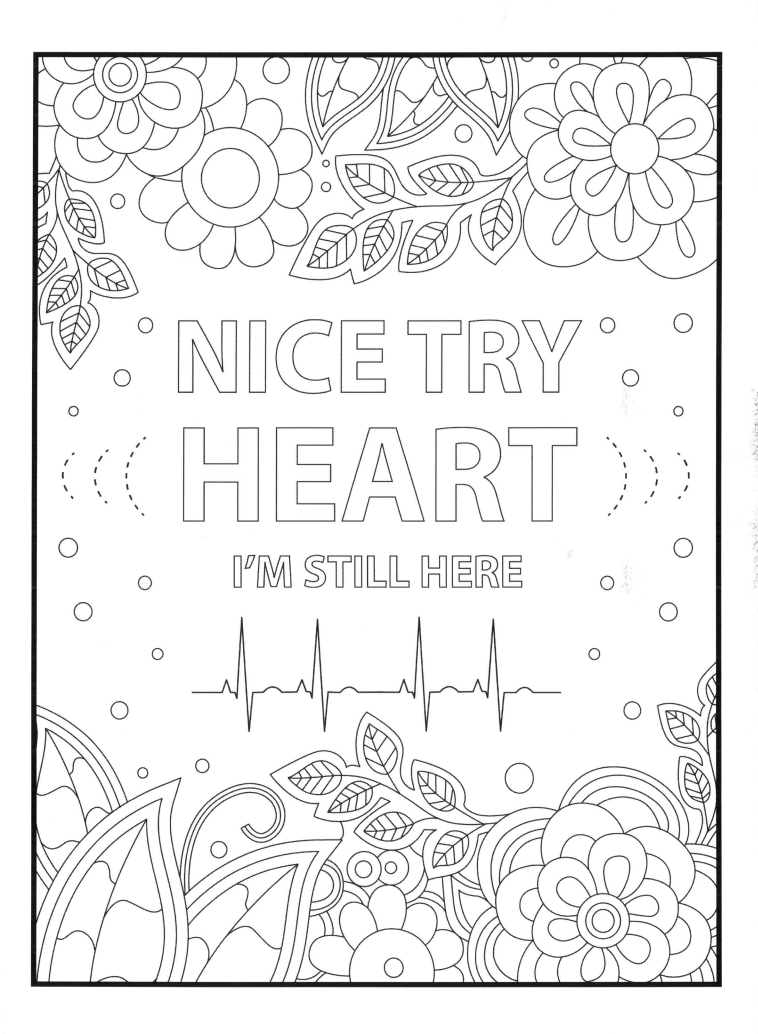

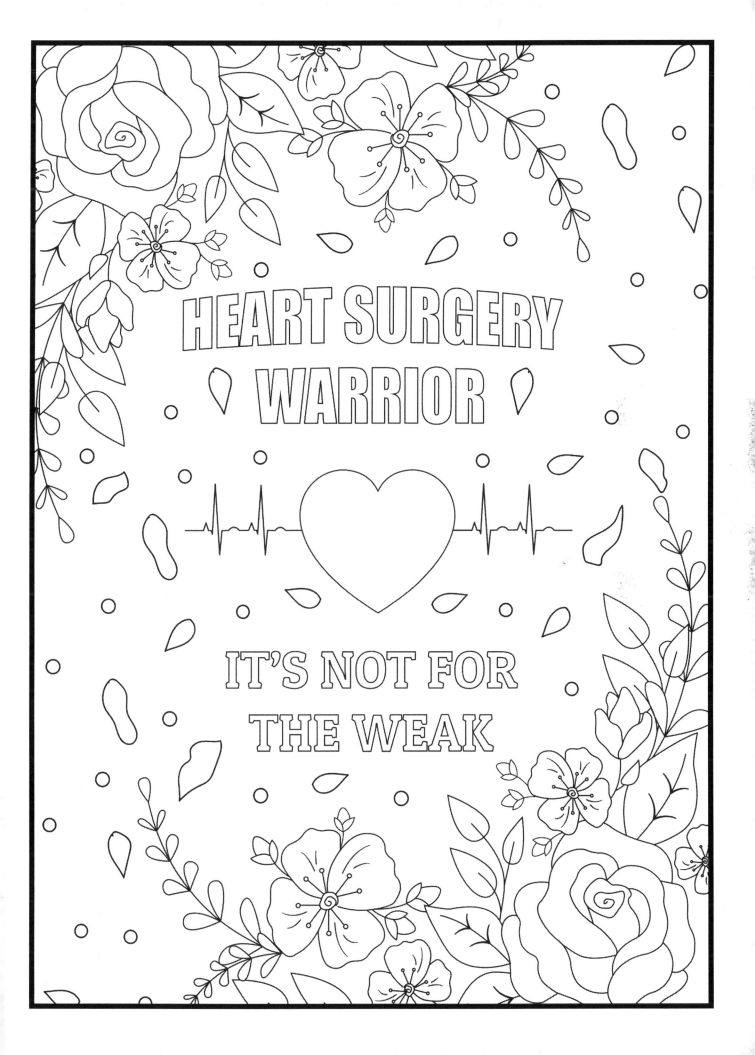

Made in the USA
Middletown, DE
13 June 2023

32533188R00027